HEALTHY AT 50

No Diets.

No Marathons.

No Gyms.

No Pain.

Just Feeling Good Every Day.

JUSTIN G. KINNEAR

Copyright © 2021 Justin G. Kinnear

All rights reserved.

ISBN: 9798701146363

WHY I WROTE THIS BOOK

I wrote this book because I recently turned 50 and had some questions. I wanted to know if turning 50 meant that it was downhill from here. Were my best years behind me? Was I ever going to feel energetic and fired up again? Was it slippers and rocking chair ahead for me?

Or, was turning 50 just another chapter. A new and exciting chapter perhaps. With my children now young men I had ever-increasing amounts of free time and space. Maybe turning 50 was a unique opening in my life.

It turned out that reaching 50 years is a unique opening. It can be a time where things become better for you because they did for me.

I decided to make some small adjustments to my daily habits and routines. Nothing too drastic, just things that I wanted to do and was willing to try for a while. These small things have changed the way I feel. They have increased my passion for living and growing as a person. That might sound a bit over the top but it's true.

In the pages that follow, I'll share with you all that I did and I'll explain why too. You can then decide if there's some part of this that could work for you, and you'll know exactly how to initiate a change.

Thanks for choosing my book. I hope you get some good ideas and find inspiration in my experience.

My very best wishes to you, my reader,

Justin G. Kinnear.

WHY YOU SHOULD READ THIS BOOK

This book will help you if you have ever felt like your best years are behind you. If you have begun to doubt if you will ever exercise again this will help. If you worry that in your later years you'll need help to do the most basic things because of your poor physical condition, it could help with that too.

If you've passed the 50 years of age milestone and are not ready to give up yet, then this book might be just right for you. And if you want to feel better, enjoy better energy levels, get some time to yourself to breathe in some fresh air, and generally feel good about your body and mind – this little book might help you to begin the journey to all that.

I'm not a doctor. I'm not a physical therapist, or nutritionist, or personal fitness coach. I'm just a regular person, like you and most other people. I don't need to be covered in muscles and don't want to be able to complete a marathon or triathlon. I want to feel good when I wake up each day. I want to be able to go up and down a flight of stairs without pain. I want to be able to get up off the sofa without emitting a loud groan. I want to be able to lift things up and down without worrying that something might snap or give.

I started simple and kept it simple. I live in the real world where life happens and things get in the way and sometimes go wrong. I don't beat myself up. I just look for a way to start up again and keep going. I am kind to myself and want to feel good about life, my health and my efforts.

This book will show you what I do and explain why I do it that way. It may be good for you too, or it may not. That, dear reader, will be determined by you.

Be kind to yourself, take your time with yourself, and be true to yourself. Let's see where these next pages take us together.

DISCLAIMER

In these pages, I share my own experiences. I describe what happened to me, what worked for me, and the effects of my choices on me.

I don't present myself in the following pages as an expert. My words should not be construed as advice or strict guidance. I am merely sharing my experiences, opinions, and outcomes.

If you have any concerns at all about whether the ideas in this book might be unsuited to your life situation or may cause you harm or injury, I urge you to consult your doctor or a similarly qualified expert before considering any of the ideas in this book.

If you do engage in any of the ideas or practices suggested in this book, you do so at your own risk and do so with your own full and voluntary intent.

CONTENTS

1 WHY WALK?

2 WALK ALONE OR WITH COMPANY?

3 CHOOSE A ROUTE

4 WALKING NEAR TRAFFIC

5 SOMETIMES THE BODY NEEDS A REST, OR DOING TOO MUCH TOO SOON

6 THE RIGHT SHOES

7 WHAT I WEAR

8 HAT AND GLASSES

9 HEADPHONES OR NOT

10 HOUSE KEYS ONLY

11 DON'T EAT FIRST

12 PUBLIC OR PRIVATE

13 TRACKING YOUR EFFORT

14 WIRE-FREE

15 WARMING-UP AND STRETCHING

16 LINKING THINGS TOGETHER
17 THE IMPORTANCE OF WATER
18 BURN ENERGY, NOT YOUR SKIN
19 CHECK YOUR FORM IS NOT DOING YOU HARM
20 THERE MAY BE PAIN
21 FOCUS ON HOW YOU FEEL
22 EATING IMMEDIATELY AFTER EXERCISE
23 DON'T OBSESS, BUT DO EAT WELL DURING THE DAY
24 EXERCISE MORE IF YOU WANT TO EAT MORE
25 CUT LOOSE WHEN YOU NEED TO
26 MY KITCHEN COLLAPSE
27 MAKE A SYSTEM (NOT A GOAL)
28 YOU CAN PUT EVERYTHING INTO A SEQUENCE
29 SWITCH TO ANOTHER REPEATABLE ROUTINE
30 EXERCISING WHEN LIFE MOVES YOU AWAY FROM HOME
31 ANY AMOUNT OF ANY EXERCISE - EVERY DAY
32 SLEEP LIKE IT'S URGENT
33 MOTIVATIONAL COLLAPSE
34 MISSING A DAY
35 WHEN ILLNESS STRIKES
36 STORMY WEATHER
37 RISKING IT ALL FOR A WALK
38 UNDOING ALL YOUR GOOD WORK

39 CONCLUSION: BE KIND TO YOURSELF
EXTRA RESOURCES FOR YOU
OTHER BOOKS BY JUSTIN G. KINNEAR
BOOKS MENTIONED IN THE TEXT

1 WHY WALK?

I am a 50-year-old male with the kind of job that involves a lot of sitting down. I used to play sports as a younger person. Football with friends in University. Five-a-side midweek football as a thirty-something until regular injuries and a general lack of fitness made me think that team sports and I were destined for separate ways.

I used to run when I was in my early twenties. I'd set off along the roads around Dublin where I live. I won't lie. It was hard on my knees. As a teenager, I was diagnosed with a knee condition that I remember as Patella Chondromalacia. This is where the muscles around the knee expand and pull the knee out of alignment, causing cartilage behind the kneecap to grind down on one side leading to some bone-on-bone action.

I took this to be something that was damaging in the long run, painful and likely to be without any lasting cure or relief. The condition seemed to define me from there.

I was officially one of those people with bad knees, and I would always have bad knees.

Every now and then, with the passing of time, I would tend to forget that I was susceptible to knee pain, and thus decide that a little jog would be good for my health. So, I'd head out and launch into a short, vigorous jog only to find myself in pain very soon again. Or I'd step onto the treadmill at home and slide the speed control up, jogging for 10 or more minutes after doing no exercise whatsoever for months if not years. It always ended the same way. Pain, frustration, and a reinforced sense that exercise and I would not be compatible ever again.

Walking? Well, that's a different story. Just about everyone can walk. And just about everyone can walk for 10 or more minutes if only they would make the time for it. I knew no matter what, if I didn't try to do too much too soon, I could manage a walk and I shouldn't expect to be in pain after it. So that's what I chose to do.

I couldn't just start running, but I could just start walking. Not silly distances. Not crazy inclines or rough terrain. Regular paths and manageable distances. No point to prove. No target to beat. No rival to race against. Just me, walking, because it should be painless and because I could just start doing it.

So can you.

2 WALK ALONE OR WITH COMPANY?

I just decided one day that I wanted to walk the very next morning to exercise. That's how it started. I was tired of feeling unhealthy, overweight, and generally guilty about my lack of activity. Almost every advert on TV made me think about my own lack of effort. I'd eat dinner with my family and spend the evening watching TV or Netflix, often climbing into bed with a sense of shame that I had done nothing to burn up calories today other than working at the computer or on the phone. So, when I decided that day that tomorrow I would fit in a walk for exercise, I never really considered the question of walking alone or with someone else. I went to bed mentally prepared to head out alone the next day.

That's precisely what I did. I got dressed in my chosen exercise clothes, put my phone in my pocket with my keys, and headed out to enjoy that first walk. That first walk then became a second, then a third and so on until it was pretty much my default way of starting the day.

Sometimes I would encounter other people along my route, mostly alone but sometimes in pairs. It never really occurred to me that it would be enjoyable to have a walking partner, mainly because I was using my walks to not only exercise but also to listen to audiobooks or podcasts.

That for me is the one thing I have come back to time and time again when I consider whether I would welcome a walking partner. It would mean I can't listen to audiobooks or podcasts and that might make the walk feel a little different. Also, sometimes I might feel that I want to walk a little faster, just to feel like I'm pushing myself a little harder. I know when I do that my heart rate increases as does my breathing rate. Trying to maintain a conversation with a partner while walking quickly just isn't realistic, so it would mean walk slower and chat, or walk faster in relative silence.

I don't have any issue with walking with a partner. It's nice every now and then to do that. I think I just prefer to walk by myself, enjoying whatever book or podcast or music I want. You should do whatever seems like the right choice for you when it comes to walking alone or with company.

3 CHOOSE A ROUTE

Starting out on the first day my plan was to walk for 5 kilometers. 5 kilometers (about 3 miles) seemed like it was enough to feel like I had walked a good distance, but not so much that I would be in pain the next day. As I said before, I have a long history of knee pain, and most of the recent instances were caused by suddenly doing lots of exercise after years of inactivity. A 5 km walk seemed like it was enough to work up a sweat without it becoming painful. It has proved to be pretty much perfect for me, at least on weekdays. It takes me roughly 55 minutes to complete 5 km so that's about the right amount of time too.

I chose my route using Google maps. I put in a destination and asked it to come up with directions on foot, and that showed me how far I might walk on the outbound leg of the walk. The return from the same point would thus yield a 5 km route.

I found a route in a loop shape that would work for me. I didn't want to walk to someplace and then turn back and walk the same journey back again. My 5 km route is a loop from my home and is a mix of flat and sloping footpaths over the 5km.

I thought about mixing up the route for variety, but it made no sense to me. If I am walking 5km and listening to a book, I'm already achieving two objectives (listen to my book, get some exercise) and I don't need a third objective (discover new things along a route). So, I walk the same route every time and I don't need to mix it up.

At the weekend I might walk a little more, sometimes extending the loop by another 30 minutes. It still doesn't cause me pain but it's a little longer and a little more of a workout. I don't need to be home for work on Saturday or Sunday so I can take a little longer on those days to complete my extended loop.

To conclude. I now have a weekday loop route (5km) and a weekend loop route (7.5km). I use the same two loops over and over. I see no great need to change the routes.

4 WALKING NEAR TRAFFIC

One thing that is worth mentioning is traffic along the route. Walking for health benefits is undermined dramatically by walking a route that has a lot of car traffic. Breathing in exhaust fumes is highly dangerous and should be avoided. We all know that exhaust fumes are harmful but sometimes when you see people walking and jogging all the time near busy roads you could be forgiven for thinking perhaps these risks are overstated. They are not overstated. Inhaling exhaust fumes from traffic is terrible for your health.

An acquaintance of mine is a NeuroScientist, and she explains in one of her books[1] how exercise plays a vital role in reenergising the body and brain by drawing in fresh oxygen. This oxygen supply fuels our muscles and our brain. The brain uses this oxygen to regenerate brain cells or neurons that have died away or need refreshing. The brain needs to do this every day along with all the other things the brain does for us to simple get through the day.

Inside your brain a substance called BDNF, or brain-derived neurotrophic factor, plays a crucial role in the generation of these new cells inside the brain. The level of BDNF in each person's brain varies, but what we do know is that people who exercise regularly appear to have higher levels of BDNF. Some scientists believe that this higher BDNF level improves memory, our capacity for learning, and better control of our emotions.

Here's the worrying part. When we exercise near a busy road and breathe in exhaust fumes, the toxic air we inhale is filled with small and dangerous particles that damage the brain's ability to produce BDNF.

When I began my new walking routine it was relatively early in the morning with very few other walkers and even fewer vehicles on the road.

Over time the level of traffic, human and vehicles, slowly started to increase. At one stage, some road works were taking place along my usual route. This caused lots of cars to idle in traffic while waiting for construction workers to wave them on their way. While this construction was ongoing, I changed my route and also changed the time of my walk so I could avoid breathing in all the fumes.

I strongly urge you not to walk and not to run near traffic. It's so bad for your health and completely undermines any possible benefit you hope to get from your activity. If you need further convincing then think about this. When researchers in the UK monitored the quality of air in a busy part of the city of London, their data showed that the levels of Nitrogen oxide that pedestrians were breathing was equivalent to smoking four cigarettes a minute.

I walk for enjoyment and for health. I hope you will too. Walking in an area and at a time of day where you are forced to breathe in very poor quality air will not be good for your health and certainly won't be enjoyable either.

Pick a time, and pick a route, that maximises the benefits to you and keeps you well away from poor quality air.

5 SOMETIMES THE BODY NEEDS A REST, OR DOING TOO MUCH TOO SOON

Things were going well, and I was managing to regularly get out for a morning walk of about 5 km each day. Then I had a brainwave. Maybe I could run a little. Just a little. Just to see how my knees might react. So, I ran a little. I'm not sure how far, not far at all. Perhaps for about 30 seconds and only at a light jogging pace. It felt ok. I was a little breathless from the change of pace from walking to jogging so I walked for the next few minutes until my breathing slowed back down to normal.

Then I did it again. I ran a little more. This time I knew after 15 or 20 seconds that today was not the day for this. I walked and slowed my breathing and went back to my original plan of completing my 5 km walk.

When I got home, I did some pre-shower exercises (push-ups, crunches, and arm weights – more about this later) and then showered. I felt fine, at least initially. Then the tightness came. At first, it was in the ligament in the back of my knee, at least that's what I think it was. It was tight and uncomfortable, pulling my leg straight when I wanted to relax it. It was tight and sore.

I tried stretching my leg, stretching my hamstrings in both legs in fact, but this only provided temporary relief at best. I knew I had overdone it.

Since about 14 years old, my knees have been a source of pain. I'm not sure why or how it began, but I suspect a combination of long periods of inactivity followed by a sudden burst of high intensity running and twisting, typically playing football in school on a concrete yard. The sudden demands on muscles and ligaments and tendons, coupled with hard pounding and twisting on a concrete yard in shoes with no cushioning whatsoever, that's a recipe for problems and it was. The muscles in my legs suddenly working hard again without any warning or warm-up, pulling and stretching tendons and ligaments out of place, pulled the alignment of my femur behind the kneecap causing heavy wear, a terrible grinding noise, and lots of pain in the joint.

Rest definitely helps. So does sports physiotherapy, especially if it involves ultrasound. The almost immediate improvement I experienced after ultrasound physiotherapy was really amazing, especially after one particular bout of pain that left me unable to carry my baby up the stairs or to get in or out of the car due to the pain I was experiencing. This particular pain came after yet another sudden and intense return to semi-competitive football in my 30s. You would think I would spot the pattern and learn my lesson but alas no.

Back to today, and the other critical factor to consider is the lack of cushioning in my walking shoes. I had returned to walking wearing my old Asics trainers. Old meaning more than 5 years for sure. What little cushioning and protection they had once offered, that was now gone. And of course, these were the shoes in which my brain figured a little run wouldn't hurt.

The tightness in my knees remained all day, especially my right knee. I had to give in and admit so to Paula and she suggested I'd have to take a rest day. I'll be honest and say it never occurred to me as an option, but it made perfect sense. In fact, after a rest day, the right knee was still a little sore, so I ended up taking two rest days.

Two days after my experimental jog I was back walking again without pain. Nice easy pace, same route as usual, just taking it easy and getting the exercise I needed.

You will have days like this, where your body is sore or aching or telling you somehow that it hurts. You should listen to it. Your body contains all the wisdom it needs to let you know when to continue and when to stop.

When your body says stop you really should. Rest, recover, and then you can go again. Also, make sure your shoes are protecting your joints with some decent cushioning.

6 THE RIGHT SHOES

Your commitment to a daily walk will depend on your shoes. If you wear shoes that are worn out, poorly fitting, or unsuitable for your walk it won't feel like something you're doing for yourself. It will feel like something you're doing TO yourself. That's like punishment. You'll eventually associate walking with pain either during or after the walk.

Do yourself a favor. Spend a little money on a decent, comfortable pair of shoes. When I started, I was wearing an old pair of Asics trainers that had served me well over the years. That was the problem. I had been wearing them for years and there was no spring left in them.

To look at them they seemed ok. The looked alright and there was still tread or grip on the sole. I wore them for the first couple of months of walking and they were ok, but one or two times, I tried to break into a light jog. Oh boy! My knees were in agony for about a week after.

My wife said to me "you have those shoes for years and years. Don't you think it's time to get some new ones? They wear out, like everything". She was right. I went to the sports store to see about some new ones. If you go there too you will be overwhelmed and maybe even confused.

First off, for walking you won't need Mo Farah marathon-strength running shoes. You're not likely to be doing that. I certainly won't. Equally, you don't want a pair of Converse All-Stars or regular tennis shoes. They don't have enough stability I would say for someone doing a regular walk.

Go for running shoes but not the most expensive ones. You don't need them. If your budget can stretch a little more than the lowest priced ones, and you can afford to buy a brand you like, and trust then why not do that. Waking up each morning to see a pair of walking shoes that you really like is the first of many joyful moments in a day. Why not make it a joyful purchase if you can afford it.

If money is a stretch, go for something that's light, comfortable on your foot and has a bit of cushion. A lack of cushioning will be hard on your knees in particular. If you don't need to scrimp then you shouldn't!

I went for a pair of Asics GT800 running shoes and I noticed the difference straight away. I don't have any pain in any joints after a walk and I've even tried a little light jog without any aftereffects. I'll stick to the walking, but it just goes to show how important it is to love your joints with shoes that cushion the blows along your daily walk.

A final word before you leave this chapter. I chose Asics shoes because this is just a personal preference of mine. When I buy running shoes, or just about anything else, I always try a variety of options until I find the one that I like best. Sometimes the best looking shoe is just not comfortable on my foot. Sometimes the most expensive shoes are just not the best choice for me, even if I had decided in my mind that I really want them.

To make a wise choice I always take my time and try a number of options. I realise that it might be sometimes difficult to get to a store and try on various shoes. You may even have to order a few pairs online, knowing you'll need to return most of them and keep the one pair that fit you best. If you spend the time picking the right ones it's time well invested in my view.

When it comes to running shoes, I have found over time that Asics shoes seem to suit me and my needs best. There are many other great shoes out there. Try them on and choose whatever you think works best for you.

Don't be guided entirely by price, by looks or by what a well meaning sales representative or amazon.com review says. They need to fit you and your needs, and feel right when you put them on. Nothing else should matter.

7 WHAT I WEAR

I walk for exercise and enjoyment. That's the sum total of what I need from it. I don't seek pain; therefore, I don't set aggressive targets for myself or push myself to walk difficult terrain. I don't seek to impress others or attract their attention. I walk for myself and for my own benefit and enjoyment.

This has a direct bearing on what I wear when I go out for my walk. I started walking in the spring when the mornings were bright and mild. I prefer to wear shorts when the weather is good so that's what I wear each day. My same pair of navy-blue Nike shorts. They have a pocket on each side, but I don't put anything in there but my house keys. They are light, comfortable and don't chafe against my skin. That's important. Don't wear anything that causes even the slightest amount of discomfort or it will start to make you associate walking with pain and discomfort.

I wear a pair of white cotton sports socks inside my Asics trainers. I've written about the shoes in another section. I could wear those tiny invisible socks that are popular these days but it's a personal choice. I find regular cotton sports socks prevent my feet from becoming itchy and irritated.

On the top, I wear a breathable exercise top, short-sleeved, and I like the Adidas Climacool clothing range. I picked up a couple on sale and they are great. They are light and don't absorb sweat as a regular t-shirt would. I don't want to be walking around and feeling self-conscious about a big dark patch of sweat on my shirt.

I choose low-key colours, like white or blue and ideally, I avoid anything with huge print or huge logos. I want to enjoy my walk without attracting attention or standing out too much. I do have a couple of bright, almost high-visibility green, exercise tops that are also breathable. I wear these if it's a little darker outside and I want to make sure others don't crash into me.

I also have a light fleece that I can wear over one of these tops just in case the temperature is a little cooler when I set off. I can wear that at the start of my walk, and if I start to feel hot, I can take that off and tie it around my waist and continue my walk without any difficulty. Layering clothes when it's colder is an old trick used by hikers and mountain walking friends and it makes sense when out walking too.

I have a light, waterproof and high visibility jacket that I can wear or bring if there's a chance of rain. It balls up into a small pouch if needed though it might be easier to just tie the arms around your waist instead of having a rolled-up ball bouncing off your hip as you walk.

Finally, when the weather is cold again, I wear a pair of plain black jogging pants. Mine are made by Nike and have little or no lettering or marks on them. I'm not planning on being an advertisement for any company and want to remain low key and not draw attention on my walk. They are not too tight, but also not too loose. I don't need any extra weight in my clothing so I chose a pair that will give me a little extra thermal insulation but won't feel heavy as I move about.

I have enough of the clothes I need that I can walk every day. If you only have one or two items of clothing that you use you will find yourself making an excuse to not walk because you have nothing to wear on a given day. Make sure you have enough. You don't need to spend a fortune, and you don't need pro gear. Find something that fits well, feels light and comfortable, and won't make you feel self-conscious or feel foolish. Plain is best when starting out.

Hang your clothes where you'll see them first thing when you wake. Why not pick out what you plan to wear the night before and then you don't even have to think about the choice. Put the clothes on and go, without any complex decision making or time wasted generating excuses to stop you heading straight out to your walk.

8 HAT AND GLASSES

Some mornings my motivation is lower than I would like. Maybe I didn't get to bed the night before as early as I hoped. Maybe I didn't sleep deeply and don't feel rested. Maybe I can hear the wind whistling outside. Maybe something in my head is trying to tell me that today, this day, the walk is a bad idea.

Other days it's more subtle. I wake up, rub my eyes and maybe even stretch a little as I lie in the final moments of sleep. I don't feel fresh. I feel ragged like I've slept in my car all night. I fear if I look in the mirror, I won't like what I see. That's probably right. Hair that screams 'BED HEAD' where it's all flat on one side and sticking up wildly on the top. That's me most mornings. And the eyes. The eyes are a bit delicate and struggling with the bright morning light.

Early on I decided I didn't want this to be anything that might get in the way of my regular walk. That's why I decided that when I walk in the morning, I wear a hat.

Usually, a cap with a peak during the milder parts of the year, and a warmer woolly hat when the weather turns colder. This way I never worry about what my hair is doing or looks like. This may seem trivial until you admit that we all care about what others think of us. If we set off with even a hint of anxiety about how we look then that's interfering with a walk. So, I put on a hat or cap and I forget all about it.

Like everything, don't wear anything on your head that will either draw attention to you or make you even mildly self-conscious. Unless of course, that's what you want. Me, I want to look like someone typical out having a walk. Nothing remarkable, nothing over the top, nothing newsworthy. Just a person going for a walk. Your average person.

Don't choose anything that doesn't fit. Seems obvious right but sometimes you might have a hat or cap that you like, maybe even really like, but it doesn't really fit and with every gust of wind off it comes. Don't wear anything that will distract from the simplicity of going for a regular walk.

I bought a plain dark blue Nike cap from a local sports store. It can be adjusted at the back. It has a tiny little logo on the front near the bottom but that's it. It's my cap that I wear so I can go straight from bed with mad hair out onto the pavement to start my walk.

Ditto the glasses. I wanted to buy some glasses that I could wear when the morning is bright, and my eyes aren't yet adjusted. I can't wait 5 or 10 more minutes while my eyes decide whether they are comfortable or not. So, I bought some polarized wraparound sunglasses online on Amazon. You buy whatever you want but, in my head, I wanted wraparound glasses like cyclists wear at the tour de France because they are lightweight, add something positive to the experience of walking, and maybe look a little bit cool. The cool part is not so crucial, but if you think your glasses make you look ridiculous then it is a problem. Buy what you like but again try not to choose something that makes you self-conscious.

If your new glasses add functionality then that's excellent. mine are polarizing and this means that they block out much of the dazzle that comes from sunlight reflecting off surfaces and boucing up towards your eyes off the road or vehicles or windows. This makes my walking experience more comfortable in very bright sun or low sun. If they add functionality such as being lightweight that's even better because you'll soon forget that you're wearing them. And if they look good and you don't flinch when you look in the mirror while wearing them – well that's a perfect blend right there.

When I'm getting ready to leave the house for my walk, the last things I put on are my headphones, then my sunglasses, then my cap. They all need to fit on and around my head comfortably. If my cap is pushing my glasses into my ears that's going to hurt. No good. If my glasses are squeezing my earphones into my head that's also no good. Try them out together and make sure they all fit together, are light and non-intrusive, and won't distract you from a good walk.

9 HEADPHONES OR NOT

I just assumed I would listen to something while I was walking. I've always enjoyed listening to audiobooks on Audible when driving across the country on business by myself. There's something nice about looking forward to the next section of an audiobook as you put on your walking gear. I suppose you could use the time to think and to just let your mind wander. I guess that's a personal choice. I prefer to listen to something.

I listen to audiobooks that I like. I think this is important and obvious. If you select an audiobook that's going to bore you, or that you are less likely to feel enthusiastic about, you end up making an association between walking and dissatisfaction. That's a really bad idea. So, pick something you like.

An author or style or subject that genuinely interests you will forge an association in your brain between walking and something that's enjoyable. You can't guarantee that the book you choose from an author you like will be enjoyable. There's an outside chance that the occasional book is not fantastic. Do your homework and get some recommendations from trusted sources.

I had a list of books and little by little I began to cross the books off the list as I walked over a prolonged period of time. I got to a place where I briefly ran out of things to listen to on my walks. I didn't spend any time replenishing my list and that was a mistake. So, as I stood in the doorway about to leave the house for my walk it was too late to choose something new. This is where podcasts can play a role.

Podcasts are highly variable. They vary in quality; in subject matter; in length and even in frequency – that is how often a new episode is released. The same basic premise applies to podcasts. Start with a topic or author/presenter that you like. The next challenge is to find a podcast that's roughly the same length as your walk.

In my case, I tend to walk each time for between 50 and 60 minutes. Finding a podcast that you like that is the right duration can be very challenging. In some instances, I have ended up listening to two 30-minute podcast episodes back-to-back. Podcasts work but they need a little planning. Audiobooks are just easier to use. Start playing when you start walking. Pause when you get home.

This brings us to the topic of the chapter. Headphones. I like to wear a cap in spring and summer or a warm woolly hat in autumn and winter. I can't imagine wearing DJ-style over-the-head headphones when I'm walking about. Also, I don't want to draw attention to myself with excessive headwear, so I prefer something more low profile. As an iPhone user, I started wearing my Apple EarPods connected by cable to my phone in my pocket. This was fine for a while until my hand somehow swung as part of my stride and dragged the wire out of the phone. It happened a few times and I didn't want to have to alter how my arms moved just to accommodate my phone and EarPods.

I did some research into wireless headphones/earphones and decided to buy a set of Beats "PowerBeats High-Performance Wireless" from the Apple store. They are a little unusual in that they are wired between the left and right earphones but wirelessly connect to the iPhone. The part that goes in my ear has a small plastic c-shaped piece that causes the earphone to grip on snugly to the ear, so it won't fall off. Having the left and right earphones snugly in place is a great feature because once they are on, I pretty much forget all about them until I am home again.

This is probably the main reason I decided not to go for the Apple AirPods – my fear of losing one of the AirPods somewhere along my walking route. AirPods owners will surely tell me I am crazy to worry about this, but I went with what I thought would work best for me.

The most important thing was decent sound quality and no wire for my arm to catch on so I can focus on walking and nothing more.

10 HOUSE KEYS ONLY

When I set off for my walk, I don't want any extra weight dragging me down. It might not seem like a big deal but when you put on your shorts or running pants or whatever you're wearing on your bottom half, the last thing you need is the weight of your bunch of house plus car plus garage plus office keys attempting to pull your clothes off as you walk.

Having to hitch up your clothes as you move is a real pain and I don't need that on my mind as I move and exercise. You want your clothes to be comfortable and somewhat loose-fitting so if you need to super tighten your tie cords so stop your pants being pulled down by your keys, you're doing it wrong.

Separate the keys you need to get back into your home from the rest of your keys, or if you're highly organised you could get an extra set of your home keys cut at the hardware store or local key cutting expert.

Watch out for new keys in your pocket though as they tend to be a little sharper and might gradually cut a little hole in your shorts/pants and then eventually your leg. Yes, this really happened.

When I leave for a walk I am focused on enjoying my walk and enjoying my book or podcast. I don't want my mind interrupted by anything else. Sunglasses digging into my head will distract my attention. Shoes rubbing or squeezing my toes or heel will distract me too. Clothes that make me feel sweaty or that restrict my movement or chafe against the skin will really bother me. I make choices so none of these things even enters my mind. That's why I don't need a huge bunch of metal keys in my pocket, sticking into my flesh or dragging my clothes down.

Minimal keys mean minimal weight. That leaves me free to enjoy my walk and focus on my book or podcast.

11 DON'T EAT FIRST

For me, what is crucial is to minimize the time between getting out of the bed and walking out the front door to start walking. Clothes and shoes on, I want to get started pretty much right away.

For a little while, I started thinking that I should maybe pre-load my body with some energy, and I had taken to eating half a banana before leaving the house. I'm pretty sure this was the opposite of helping.

When you wake up and get straight to walking, the exercise involved in using the muscles around your body immediately looks for an energy source. It's likely to have been 6 or more hours since you last ate so the chances are your body will attempt to consume resources stored around your body as fat. This is good. Very good. Your extra fat is designed for that purpose so as you exercise in the morning, your body slowly, gently, carefully consumes some of this fat.

If you eat before you leave the house for your walk, that's what your body will absorb. Not the fat but the half banana because it's right there in your stomach and easier to access.

It is a good idea to have some water before you go. Me, I drink about half a glass of water out of my water filter jug. No reason. I just made it a habit to have water in the filter jug at room temperature on the kitchen table and a glass right next to it. I walk down the stairs ready to walk, nip into the kitchen to grab my keys, pour and drink half a glass of water at room temperature, and then quietly slip out of the house and on to my walk.

12 PUBLIC OR PRIVATE

I have often heard it said that sharing a goal with others makes the commitment stronger. This might be true for some things but I'm not sure that I agree that public sharing helps here. I say that for two reasons. The first, my walk every day is not really a goal. Instead, it's more like a routine or system that I have developed for myself. Its purpose is to create an activity that I look forward to and that provides a health benefit to me and me alone. Sharing what I am doing beyond say my immediate family doesn't make much sense to me. Sharing with the immediate family does, especially if a member of the household is wondering who is leaving the house at 7 am.

The second reason I have for not sharing that I walk or why is that I feel it's nobody else's business. I walk for me, for my own enjoyment and that's it. I can't think of a good reason to mention my routine to friends. Maybe they will offer to join me, but that's something I don't necessarily want. Maybe they will offer me advice about routes or ask me about my personal best for 5 km. Those conversations are also something I don't want.

I make one exception about sharing and that's this book. My walking works for me as an individual, a private individual. Maybe there's someone out there just like me who is wondering about starting up some light exercise and wonders if they have the willpower to stick with it.

If this book can provide some encouragement to even one person like me then it will have been worth sharing my experience with you the readers. I don't share to set myself up as some role model or ideal example. I'm just a regular person who started a routine and stuck with it because it was enjoyable and not too difficult, and it made me feel good.

13 TRACKING YOUR EFFORT

I like the way that I look forward to exercising. I don't have a negative relationship with my walk, or my shoes, or some other aspect of the activity that is uncomfortable, or worse, painful. That would make no sense to me. That's why I also don't obsess about tracking myself when I exercise.

It's not true to say that I don't track my activity. I do. At least, one of my devices does that for me. I started out walking with my iPhone X in the pocket of my shorts. I wore my EarPods wired headphones plugged into the iPhone and it was fine to begin with. The health app on the phone seemed to know I was walking or running or going up or down stairs. It did that without any prompting from me, which is both amazing and a little intrusive.

Anyway, when I'd walk it would usually last about an hour. My aim was to identify a route of approximately 5 kilometers (about 3 miles) that I could walk each day. I found out that the route I chose took about 55 minutes to complete each time. The phone would track and tell me that information and I have to say I never paid much attention to it.

The annoying saga of my swinging arm catching and pulling out the headphone cable (covered in another chapter) caused me to initially switch to wireless earphones. This was an excellent idea in hindsight. The weight of the phone also made me contemplate leaving it at home and replacing it with an apple watch. This was also a good idea since it's a lot lighter than the phone, but there are some considerations.

My apple watch is obsessed with telling me things about my 'performance'. I probably could find and turn off some of these settings, but inertia and no real inconvenience cause me to leave things as they are. The watch tells me when I have completed 1 km of my walk and also how long that took. Yes, my pace per kilometer is being tracked and relayed to me by my watch. Good to know I suppose but it's not what drives me. I don't want to push harder than is enjoyable. The watch reminds me of my pace again at 2 km, and then at 3 km. You see what's happening.

My watch also wants to remind me to stand if I have been sitting a long time and this is useful. I have experienced some back and neck pain in the past after long bouts of sitting in front of the computer. An occasional reminder to get up and move about can be very timely indeed.

I am also reminded to breathe by my watch and while the idea is well intentioned, sometimes the moment it chooses to remind me is laughably inappropriate. I will say no more.

So, it's good to have some data on my exercise but mainly so I know I have completed 5 km. This is less of an issue outdoors because I know the route I walk and it will be 5 km. If the weather is bad or the day has been a challenge and I could not get outside, the watch will help me while I'm walking on the exercise machine to ensure I do get a 5 km walk.

Bizarrely while my iPhone X knows that I'm moving and will track my distance travelled automatically, my watch prefers to be notified that I am about to exercise. This seems odd to me but that's how it is. Once or twice it has asked me if I am working out and then reveals that it has been tracking my movement in the background, just in case I forgot to inform my watch of my work out!

The upshot of all this is that I have a relaxed relationship with tracking. I don't need to know if I'm getting faster or my heart is beating faster. I get most of the value from the watch through books and podcasts and the wireless link to my headphones.

I don't want to be taunted or tormented by my data telling me I should be doing better and that I am failing at exercising. I set the agenda and the purpose and I'm happy with the performance data as courtesy information. It means no more than that to me.

14 WIRE-FREE

It's not a big deal but I try to avoid any wires running from one place to another around my body while I'm exercising. You'd be surprised how annoying it can be for your hand to routinely catch in your headphone cable while you're out walking, yanking it out of your phone and disturbing the nice flow you had going at that moment.

A phone in a pouch strapped to your arm, connected to your earphones via a cable, seems like it could be a simple solution to music on the go but the mere act of putting more weight on one arm causes a subtle imbalance and is one more subconscious thing for your brain to worry about.

I resisted it for a while, but I eventually got rid of the cabled earphones and got some wireless Bluetooth earphones and that stopped me thinking about getting my hand caught as I walked. I literally never think about it since.

I also stopped bringing my iPhone with me and now just use an Apple watch. You don't have to use an Apple watch of course but the idea is not to lug around a 6-ounce iPhone (mine is an X) in the pocket of your shorts or joggers or strapped to your arm. Instead, my Apple watch weighs 1.7 ounces, so that's better and almost unnoticeable. Alternatively, a cheap Bluetooth MP3 player or radio weighing less than an ounce would also work just great.

Keep the weight of whatever media source you're using to a minimum and get rid of any trailing cables or wires so you can just get on with a great walk and enjoy whatever you're listening to without an annoying interruption every time your swinging arm catches the wire and yanks it out of place.

15 WARMING-UP AND STRETCHING

I used to think I should stretch before I walk. It seemed logical to me to spend a few minutes warming up muscles, stretching and rotating and all that before heading out. Here's what I found to be true for me. The times I spent stretching made no material difference to my walk, my enjoyment of that walk, or my likelihood to attract or avoid injuries.

I also found the time I spent stretching beforehand felt like an inconvenience. It was delaying me from starting my walk.

This was important because anything that has the potential to delay the walk or to plant a seed of doubt about whether I really wanted to go walking, well that's just not helpful to me. So, I made a call to not bother with stretches beforehand.

The deal I made with myself is this. The alarm goes off and I slide out of bed and into the clothes laid out the night before. Watch on. Wireless headphones on. Sunglasses on. Hat on. Drink a small glass of water in the kitchen. Grab my house keys. Gently open and then close the front door after me. Begin walking nice and gently.

Here's what I figure. If I don't set off like I'm competing in the Olympics, my body will gradually and gently come up to temperature. The muscles will gently stretch and flex and work as intended. My breathing and blood flow will do what it already knows how to do.

As long as I don't begin my walk like a maniac, there's no real need for me to warm up or stretch beforehand. Stretching delays the walk, introduces the potential for excuses and resistance, and seems to be unnecessary to me.

What's more interesting is the time right after I get back home after the walk. The way I see it, my body is fully warmed up and stretchy and this seems like a perfect time for some exercises before the shower. I'm sweaty already so why not extract one last opportunity before the clothes go into the laundry basket and I go into the shower.

This is why I do my push-ups, crunches and arm/chest exercises at this point. It makes perfect sense to me so that's why I do it in this order. To me, this is the best place for stretches and rotations and whatever else I feel like doing before getting into the shower.

I usually spend about 10 minutes doing exercises right outside my shower, then off with the sweaty workout clothes and into the shower. To me, this is my ideal sequence and the ideal place for exercises and stretches in my routine.

16 LINKING THINGS TOGETHER

I'm the kind of person who has always struggled to stick with new habits. I want to succeed. I want to drop an old behaviour that doesn't serve me well any longer and replace it with a new behaviour. My intentions are good, but my follow-through isn't always brilliant. My pattern, up to now, has been to start well and succeed for a few days, before falling back into old behaviours and telling myself it's not my fault. The excuses come easily and make reasonable sense, but they are just excuses. Sometimes I really beat myself up about not sticking with my new habits and other times I secretly shrug my shoulders as if to say "what did you expect? You never stick with it"

That's why the book Tiny Habits[2] by B.J. Fogg was such a big help to me. B.J.'s book helped me to see that there are a few different facets to forming a new habit, one of which is creating a routine that provides a visual reminder to strengthen the habit.

For me, this has changed my commitment to exercise and walking completely and made it easier to stick with the behaviours I want. Here's what I do.

Every time I walk, I get sweaty which is good. Sweaty means I'll need to take a shower. Between walking and stepping into the shower I place a mini workout routine with just three parts.

I start with push-ups on the floor right outside the shower. Initially, I could manage just 5 push-ups because I was out of shape, but that can increase over time and it has increased.

Next, I do crunches on the floor right outside the shower. I am trying to work the muscles in my core and again I start small. I began by watching a video on how to do crunches at home and the guidance was for 14 gentle crunches. This worked for me and I can do more now that my muscles can handle a bit more of a workout.

I finish with my weights. I have two 5 kg weights on the floor where I am working out and I do three different exercises with the weights. The specifics of my pre-shower exercises are at the back of the book if you want to try them for yourself.

Here's the thing. These exercises help to balance out the benefit of the walk. When I walk my lungs and legs and heart and skin all get some benefit but my arms and upper body not as much. So, these three exercises help me to spread the benefit a bit wider once I get home and all the blood and oxygen is pumping around the body and I'm nicely warmed up.

It's important that I can do these exercises in a relatively short amount of time before I hit the shower. Together they take less than 10 minutes, and they work all the other muscles enough that it's worth sticking with the little routine. Each time I walk I exercise. The two routines are locked together. That's the idea I took from B.J. Fogg's great book, and there are other ideas but more about that later.

It's also important that these exercises are private. I don't need or want anyone else knowing all about my pre-shower routine. I am slowly and steadily exercising. I am slowly and steadily improving my health. I am slowly and steadily working muscles and I know that it's going to take time before I notice any change in my muscle tone. To be clear, I'm not looking to build muscle and get ripped. I'm just looking to exercise a bit more than the walk provides.

From time to time, I have added some extra little routines on top of these three exercises, but I don't do that all the time. These three are my core exercises and whenever I walk I do these three.

I now knew that I was forming a new habit sequence. Dress. Water. Walk. Water. Push-ups. Crunches. Weights. Undress. Shower. And I was able to stick with it. For a long time. Without any real effort, I had made this my way of starting the day. I now also knew I couldn't get push-ups and crunches into the time that it took the shower to warm up but now realised this was irrelevant. The exercise while warmed-up idea had taken root and the shower could wait a few more minutes.

I started each of these with 5 repetitions, taking care to go slowly and carefully and not trigger a muscle injury due to over-zealous diving in. I gradually built-up to 15 of each and that is a good balance for me. The various muscles feel like they have had a stretch and it delays me from the shower by about 10 minutes. Any longer and I can start to worry about my working day being knocked off course.

The space between the walk and the shower is really magic because it's part of an established routine. Add anything into this space (brushing your teeth for example) and it instantly becomes a strong part of your daily habit.

The space between your head and your hips is also magic. It's your core. This area is the source of so much strength in the body and protects the vital organs.

Anything you can do to build even a little more strength in your arms, chest, abdomen, back and anywhere connected to these areas will help you feel strong and healthy.

All you are doing here is delaying the shower and it's a golden opportunity to add one or two little extras for no real cost.

I still add the occasional extra exercise in here, but my holy trio of push-ups, crunches and arm weights follow just about every walk I take and I barely notice the time and effort to complete them.

Try and fit some core exercises into the magic space before you hit the shower.

17 THE IMPORTANCE OF WATER

I know that you know this. Water is really important to your body and brain. It's the stuff that so much of the body is made from, and it's literally what sustains us every day. But we don't always drink enough of it.

Here's my simple way of looking at it. If I am going out for a walk that will last up to an hour, I consider the weather and how much I think I might sweat. If it's really warm or I think I'll sweat a fair bit, I'll definitely bring water with me.

If it's cooler or more winter-like conditions I won't bring water, but I'll drink a half glass of water before I leave the house for my walk. I won't drink more than that because I don't want to be bursting for a pee 30 minutes later, so a half-glass works well for me.

When I get home the first thing I do when I get into the house is drink some more water. I'm not going to tell you to down a specific amount. I don't bother setting myself some target of how much to drink. I drink about a half-glass again but if I'm still thirsty I drink some more. It's that simple.

Later, after a shower and some exercises, the body is warm from the shower and readjusting to the house temperature and so I'll carry a water bottle with me from room to room in case I'm feeling a little thirsty. It's not so easy to know that you are mildly dehydrated after exercise so "drink when you are thirsty" is as simple a rule as you can muster.

I do like a coffee later and it's worth remembering that coffee has a dehydrating effect on the body, like many other things. Keep drinking the water if you continue to feel like you might need it.

Some people advocate examining your urine, by eye of course, and if it's really dark then you need to drink more water. Another example of the amazing ways that this is not so difficult to figure out. The body is built to tell you to stop walking (knee pain), drink more water (dark urine), eat something (rumbling stomach) and so on.

Heed the body, respect the body, feed it water when it needs.

And the brain. If you think you can go along fine without water, just remember that your brain suffers too when you're dehydrated. A small drop in water level in the body might not sound too serious, but when the brain is one of the largest users of oxygen in the entire body it suddenly sounds like a bad idea to starve your brain of one of the main sources of oxygen.

Water before you exercise, and water after you exercise. Start there. Then make sure to have water available all through the day for when you need it. Having a coffee, have some water too. Having lunch. Have some water too.

Finally, your kidneys may thank you for making sure you get all the water you need. Your kidneys rely on a good supply of water to help them flush out stuff that the body doesn't need. Not enough water means not enough flushing. You don't want that stuff inside you that should be outside you.

Respect your body by making sure you give it the water it needs, but don't obsess about it.

18 BURN ENERGY, NOT YOUR SKIN

If you are lucky, some of the days you set off for a walk will be fine days. Nice weather. Dry with maybe a gentle breeze is ideal. Some days will be warmer than that and you might imagine how nice it will be to walk and get a tan at the same time.

Some people presume that the sun's intensity is not so strong in the morning, for example, and don't worry about the chance of being burned by the sun as you walk. Me, I'm not taking that chance. I walk to feel good, to give my body an opportunity to exercise and burn up some energy while also creating new energy. What I don't want is to burn my skin in the process.

I just sidestep this issue altogether and make it so that if the weather is warm and bright and there's even an outside chance of sunburn, no matter how mild, I'll apply some sun protection to my exposed skin before I leave. I leave my SPF50 spray right where I can see it so when I am putting on my walking clothes it's no big deal to spray my arms, legs, back of my neck and ears and anywhere else that might be struck by the sun. Remember I am wearing sunglasses and a cap, so my face is well protected just about all the time, all the days.

If the purpose of the walk is to feel healthier, why would you introduce the possibility that your walk might be the source of some future skin problem because you wouldn't spend 30 seconds spraying your arms and legs with sun protection?

Show some love for yourself by protecting yourself on those days where it really is necessary.

19 CHECK YOUR FORM IS NOT DOING YOU HARM

Form is a word that athletes, physiotherapists, and those who are interested in exercise use when assessing how a person's posture is aligned with the needs of a particular activity. For example, if you wanted to set off on a light run or a fast sprint, a trainer or physio watching your movement could assess if you were demonstrating the right form for the run or sprint. They would look at the angle of your back, which part of your foot was striking the ground, how high your knees come up, what your arms are doing when you run, and so on.

Why are they looking at this form? Well, like anything, there's no point in doing the activity if it results in harm to you instead of the intended benefit. Assessing form allows a coach or physio to make sure that you get the benefit from the activity without doing some longer-term damage.

Surprisingly, everything from a simple push-up to a long-distance run will benefit from making sure that your form is right. A few minutes spent finding out how an exercise should be done can help to prevent long-term problems with muscles and bones.

There are a few different options here, the most expensive ones being to join a gym or engage a personal trainer or even visiting a sports physiotherapist for advice. It might be strange to visit a physiotherapist before problems occur though, as they are usually visited by people that have already done some damage or are experiencing pain, speaking from personal experience.

I don't want to join a gym or engage a personal trainer, so I went for the zero-cost option to check my form. YouTube. I have one important rule when it comes to using YouTube for advice. Never trust a single video. So, I watched a heap of videos about form, usually focusing on one activity at a time. Yes, there are videos about walking form. I found that from time to time I would experience some pain in my lower back. Videos helped me to work out why the walking was making my back sore and what to do to prevent it. Same for pushups, crunches, and various other forms of exercise I like to do after my walk.

I have learned a lot about how the body works, and why pain sometimes follows exercise even when taking things easy. Nowadays if I'm going to take on a new activity, I'll assume my instinctive form will be wrong and I go and find out what is the best way to approach it. It has saved me pain, helped me heal the pain I had from bad technique, and also helped me to develop a realistic assessment of my instincts when it comes to exercising.

In order to do it right, it always makes sense to spend some time to learn how to do it right. This is a good maxim for most things.

20 THERE MAY BE PAIN

Every now and then, despite my very best efforts to avoid pain, some part of my body becomes a source of pain. It could be something minor, such as irritation between my toes. Or it could be something more troublesome, such as a nagging pain in the lower back or in the knee joint. The sensible thing to do anytime pain arrives is to take a break from exercise and instead take a rest day.

On a rest day, I avoid any strenuous activity or exercise and really try to protect the part of the body that hurts. If there is still some pain the day after a rest day I'll simply take another rest day. This is often enough and a day or two after resting things feel normal again and I gently resume my routine.

Sometimes this is not the case. After a number of days away from exercise, I may still feel pain in a part of the body. When I was younger, I used to ignore these pain signals and just push on, telling myself that I could somehow overpower the pain with a mix of positive thinking and sheer force of will. That never worked out well for me. Nowadays when I experience pain that lasts longer than a few days I make a choice in my mind. Should I see my doctor or my chiropractor?

When I speak about my chiropractor, I'm conscious that it possibly makes me sound like a Beverley Hills celebrity. I say my chiropractor because, though there are many chiropractors available, I have found one that really works for me and with whom I have a trusting and candid dialogue. He expects me to be completely honest with him and I expect him to be the same with me. It really works as a relationship.

I have been to many physiotherapists over the years but very few could help me with the pain I experienced at the time. My chiropractor seems to be able to identify the causes of pain and can manipulate me in a way that allows me to walk out feeling better than I did when I walked in 20 minutes before.

The point I am laboring here is simple. Don't ignore pain. If it's something to do with muscles or the body's bone structure, it's worth paying a visit to a chiropractor for an assessment or some simple manipulation.

If it's something else, it may require a conversation with your doctor.

Ignoring pain is something many men do and it's not smart, especially for pain that persists for a number of days.

21 FOCUS ON HOW YOU FEEL

As a younger person, I had many experiences of sport and exercise that made me associate these kinds of activities with pain, suffering and many other negative feelings. I enjoyed sport for sure, especially when it was fun and taking place with friends.

When sport and physical activity is a thing that makes us feel bad, because we don't make the team, or because I can't climb a flight of stairs afterwards, that's not ideal. It's hard to think of any other human endeavor we choose to engage in that results in us feeling rejected, dejected, depressed or in extreme pain.

I know many people see sport as a way of proving something about themselves to themselves. Whatever. Each person should be free to do whatever they want when it comes to how they relate to sport and exercise.

Where others obsess about personal best scores for how long it takes to run or walk a distance, or how hard they pushed themselves in the gym, or how many pounds of weight they lost over a week, I don't. I don't concern myself with all that stuff, at least not primarily. At the age of 50, I need to show some respect for my body and my brain.

Common sense alone tells me that a 50-year-old body responds differently to strain and pain than a 20-year-old body can. I need to be more measured, more intelligent, and more respectful about what I expose my body to when it comes to exercise.

Instead of obsessing about whether I am getting faster, stronger, lighter and all that I instead focus on how I feel. Do I feel healthier, more able to get up off the couch without the audible groan? Can I walk farther without feeling breathless, or climb stairs with ease, or lift heavy items up and down in the Garage where I store my tools? I am exercising for a better quality of life and more ease in living.

I want to lose some extra weight that I have accumulated. That's obvious. I don't need to obsess about it though and get it done in 4 weeks solid. I know it took some time to add on that extra weight so it might take time and patience to lose the extra weight and keep it off. If I can remodel my habits over time so that I improve my health and how I feel about myself then that's the way I'm going to do it.

Pushing yourself really hard will put your body under strain. It's not likely to produce any lasting benefit nor are you likely to create new healthier habits to replace old unhealthy habits. You'll learn that these diets and exercise bursts never work, at least that's the lesson you'll take from it all. You'll also develop a subtle negative association, that exercise is something you do to yourself when you are a failure.

I want exercise in my life, but I want it to be something that works for me, and with me. I want exercise to be something that I enjoy, that is flexible and can bend according to what's going on in each week, and that I look forward to doing whenever I can, no matter how little time I have or where I may be.

This kind of relationship with exercise makes me feel healthy and makes me appreciate every little way that exercise does good for my body and brain. I focus on how exercise makes me feel positive, and don't allow myself to use exercise as a way to bring pain and suffering into my week.

Exercise is a source of good feelings for me and that's the way I want it to be.

22 EATING IMMEDIATELY AFTER EXERCISE

In summary, I don't do it. When I get back home or finish a walk on the treadmill if the weather is bad, I drink water. Not too much. Just enough to not feel parched any longer. I don't want too much water sloshing around inside me right after I exercise. I head for the shower, spending a few minutes between ending the walk and hitting the shower on some simple exercises that I like. I'll often do some push-ups, some gentle and slow weight exercises with the dumbbells, and some crunches for the middle section around the belly. I don't want a load of food in there, so I wait.

Usually, after I shower and get dressed, I am calm again and my pulse and breathing have returned to normal. My heart is not racing, and my mind is not craving food. By going without food straight away after exercise, I get more benefit from the body recovering from the walk and exercises. The body will draw from the resources in and around my body, which is really what I want to happen.

Don't be stupid about this though. If you have not eaten much in the last 8-10 hours and you overdo it with your walk or exercise you may be low on bodily reserves of energy and it could cause you to get lightheaded or woozy.

Be careful. Listen to your body. If you need something to eat, then eat. Try not to eat too much too close to heading out, otherwise your body will want to divert blood to the stomach to break down what you ate. Your muscles and lungs also need to use this blood. This causes an internal tension that you and your body don't need.

23 DON'T OBSESS, BUT DO EAT WELL DURING THE DAY

For me, at 50 years of age, exercise is something I use to keep myself feeling good. Too many times I have bent over to pick something up off the lawn and experienced pain and stiffness in various parts of my body. Too many times I have found myself letting out a grunt when trying to get up after a bout of watching Netflix on the TV. I may be 50 but I shouldn't feel like I am 100. I'm certain I should not feel sore after kneeling down to inflate my car tires, but sometimes in the past I did feel sore. I want to feel good and that's why I exercise. Exercise keeps everything moving and working and healthy.

On the other hand, I am not over-focused on my weight or appearance. I don't have a target weight. That's something I could end up obsessing over and this would ruin the good feeling that exercise brings me. I don't want to sit in a restaurant or around the kitchen table with my family and be consciously totting up calories and seeing food as a source of danger to my weight plans.

I try to strike a balance when it comes to food. We all know that too much of anything is not good, and we also all know that certain kinds of foods while tasting great are probably not going to help as we try to get and stay healthy. I don't obsess about what I eat or what my family eats but I am trying to strike a balance so that we all have the best chance to feel healthy and have a healthy relationship with food.

One of the simplest things I do when it comes to eating well after exercising is to think about the effort my body will need to expend to break down what I eat. It goes without saying that foods that have required a great deal of processing in a factory will almost certainly need a fair bit of processing in the body too. Foods that look and taste like they did when they were harvested by human hands will generally require less processing effort by the body.

Remember the body has a limit to all the things it can do each day. That's why we need sleep and food and exercise to regenerate energy. So even something as small as making a choice to have fruit for dessert rather than cake or ice cream is a big help to the body.

So, without obsessing about what I eat, if exercise does indeed make you feel good then maybe it's time to consider if the things you eat, and the amount you eat, during the day are undoing all the wonderful benefits that exercise brings to the brain and body.

24 EXERCISE MORE IF YOU WANT TO EAT MORE

It's a simple equation. The body tries to keep energy in balance. In order to create energy, it must consume energy. You know that there is such a thing as a recommended daily intake of various food types and vitamins. That's because we only need a certain amount of those things each day if it is indeed a typical day.

If it's not a typical day, for example a celebration or a holiday or Superbowl Sunday or something like that, we might find ourselves eating and drinking more than we would normally. That's understandable. Just know that the body doesn't know it's a special day and is not really sure what to do with all the extra food and drink you ingest. It will try to use up some of it in the usual way, but some of what you take on board is not needed right now and might be passed back out as waste. Some however might also be stored onboard, in the form of body fat. Keep eating and drinking more than your body needs and you know where this is going.

Keeping a healthy respect for food and what the body actually needs in the front of your mind will definitely help. Another thing that will help is recognising that exercise will consume some of these calories too. Let's be careful here though. It's not a good idea to wake up suddenly and feel guilty about the birthday cake or bowl of popcorn you ate last night, jump out of the bed and immediately launch into an over-the-top walk or run that is way more demanding than your body is used to. This will cause you pain and you'll regress instead of progress.

If you are tempted not to go for a walk, this might be the morning that a walk is very much to be welcomed. If you normally walk for 50 minutes why not walk for an extra 10, or even pick up the pace a little bit. Not enough to cause pain but enough to create a little more burn of energy.

If you want to eat more then you will need to exercise a little more to keep things somewhat balanced. If you want to eat more all the time, then exercise might not help you here.

Once again, the point here is not to make exercise a thing you do to yourself because you have been naughty. Exercise is a wonderful gift that you give to yourself, to enjoy feeling alive and feeling grateful for the ability to move and breathe and observe and interact with the world.

Don't overdo it with the food and drink more than you should, and keep in mind the need to keep things in balance when it comes to the food your body needs, and the importance of exercise in playing its part in keeping the body and brain in balance.

25 CUT LOOSE WHEN YOU NEED TO

Every now and then there will be some special occasion. A birthday, an anniversary, a promotion, or any number of other reasons to celebrate. This can be a source of real tension as you imagine all the good work you've done evaporating under a mountain of ice cream cake and cold beer or some other irresistible treat that you have been carefully avoiding.

While this tension, and the accompanying guilt, might be well-founded it is important to remember that exercise is not the enemy. Exercise is not in your life to ruin your life or to prevent you from ever enjoying yourself again. If that's where exercise now sits it might be time to reassess why you are exercising at all, at least from my perspective.

If you have a special occasion, and there might not be too many of them right now, why not allow yourself to cut loose and enjoy the moment. Chances are you might regret being a wet towel in the middle of everyone else's good feelings, and would it really kill you to take a night off every now and then.

I'm all for cutting loose on one condition. That you remember that everything must return to balance. So the more you eat and drink, the more you'll be out of balance for a few days. Why not make a deal with yourself to enjoy the occasion but to keep a lid on how much you eat and drink. Have a burger but don't have three burgers. Have a beer but don't drink all the beers.

I like to hang my exercise gear out on display just before I go out to an occasion like this. It sends me a powerful visual reminder that I shouldn't go too crazy with the food and drink, not least because I'll be wearing these clothes tomorrow and will need to work harder to get back in balance.

Enjoy yourself but remember that you need to bring things back into balance as soon as you can. Don't let exercise be the enemy of good times, or become the thing that others perceive to be the reason why you are no fun anymore. That's not what exercise should mean in anyone's life.

26 MY KITCHEN COLLAPSE

In hindsight, it was stupid of me, but at the time I felt it was a reasonable thing to do. Let me go back to the start. About 4 weeks after I started my new relationship with a daily walk I decided to cut back on sugar and carbohydrates. I really felt that, between cake and biscuits and pasta and bread and breakfast cereal, I had way too much carbohydrate in my diet. Walking would help me to feel healthier but surely cutting back on this sugar/carbohydrate-based stuff would help too.

So, I decided one day, after gradually eating less and less of the carbohydrates that were normal for me, that it would be a sugar-free day. All was fine, and again the next day with no sugar there was no real issue. I think it was the third day without any sugar intake when I woke as normal for my walk. I got dressed and went down to the kitchen for my pre-walk water. About half a glass was all I usually drank, turned on the headphones and set my watch and off I went, grabbing my keys on the way out.

The walk was great, the weather lovely, and after about 50 minutes I was back home. I walked into the kitchen. Everyone else was still in bed and the house was quiet. I went to pour myself a glass of water from the filter jug. I moved it from one countertop to another in front of me and set it down.

I woke with a strange feeling. The side of my face felt cold and the feeling of something rough against my cheek was unexpected. I opened my eyes and realised I was lying on the tiles in the kitchen. I had hit the floor. Collapsed. Passed out. Fainted. Whatever. I had hit the deck.

I got to my feet, drank the water I now realised I had not drunk and went to the bathroom to inspect my face. Aside from a slight graze on my cheek just under my left eye, there were no other injuries to report. I was lucky. I suspect I must have gently slumped down onto the ceramic tiles, otherwise, I reckon I would have hurt myself more seriously.

What happened? My guess is cutting out sugar so quickly and so completely really drained me of energy reserves. My walk was fine. Normal. But it probably used up the last extra energy I had available and when I got home, a mix of being energy depleted and slightly dehydrated made for a dangerously low ability for the body to regulate itself, so it shut down. I went into standby temporarily, while the muscles recovered from the exertion of the walk. That's my guess.

Do some exercise is my mantra. No matter how small. Do something to keep healthy and keep active. I don't advocate for over-the-top exercise or pushing things to the max. Some people want and need to do that. That's their goal. Me, I want to be healthy and not out of breath doing simple things. It's a good idea to watch what you eat, especially things that you eat a lot of, or that you know are not very healthy. Be careful though.

Completely eliminating the things the body needs a basic level of to function and regulate is risky. If you're going to cut stuff out, and you think there could be a knock-on effect, why not run it by your doctor or another medical professional. The body is clever, designed to self-manage and self-heal within limits, but it also needs you to fuel it properly. Make sure you don't run out of fuel like I did, in a rush to purify yourself.

27 MAKE A SYSTEM (NOT A GOAL)

We love goals these days. From an early age, young people are taught about the importance of having a goal. Goals, they say, give direction to our efforts. They allow us to make the leap from where we are to where we want to be and feel good about ourselves.

There's one shortcoming with the way we use goals. Once we achieve our goal, we become almost immediately unsatisfied with that and want to set a new goal. Ever bought something that you really, really wanted. Maybe you waited a long time and had to save for ages. Sadly, things rarely feel as satisfying as we imagined after all that build-up.

Imagine you want to be able to run for 30 minutes straight, or maybe you want to reach your target weight of 70 kilos. Good for you. So you decide to get to work, hitting the road every day or watching what you eat every mealtime until finally, you reach your goal. If you're like most people you will likely have shared your goal with a few friends, so there's a certain satisfaction in sharing your success with them too. Then what?

Well once the goal is achieved there's either an almost-immediate re-appraisal of the situation to set a new goal. You can't sit on your backside and just do nothing now, can you? Or maybe you can take a break, a well-earned break, only to find some of that hard-earned success has quickly slipped away and you're now steadily sliding back to where you started.

This is a challenge I have experienced with goals, and I can't be the only one. Don't get me wrong here. I admire people who set goals and I think we should all be aiming for something that is good for us and gives us a better quality of life. My issue is with the focus on the finish line. That is what the achievement of a goal represents to me.

Instead of goals, I think of the same basic idea here. I want to be able to run for a certain time or distance or want to weigh a certain weight. The trap is to fixate on the end result when what I find works better is to slowly and carefully create new habits and routines that will reshape my behaviour, so the goal emerges organically. I'd rather develop a habit of getting up each day and making the same healthy breakfast over say a 4-week period than obsessively weighing myself each morning.

The key is the routine, and not the outcome. Likewise, if the way to increase my running capability is to run regularly, then the habits I establish to increase my chances of a regular run are more important than the moment when I can run 30 minutes straight.

So, I change my habits in order to change my outcomes and to change my habits I create systems. A system is a pattern of behaviour that I teach myself to follow each day. I'll have the odd day where I deviate but because my system is a well-worn path, I can get back on track easily.

One of the best ways of creating systems is to bundle actions together. For example, I always brush my teeth before I get into bed, so why not add 2 minutes of exercise every night right before brushing my teeth. It's as simple as that. Or why not park your car a little distance from the shop so you get a short walk every time you go shopping. Why not drink a glass of water with each cup of coffee.

Bundling actions into a system means you shape a new habit or routine. Then when you do hit your goal, if it matters to you, you can just keep going with your system to maintain your success. You don't feel the "right, what do I do now?" feeling that so many people feel when they hit their goal, because it's not all about the goal. It's all about systems.

I tip my hat to Scott Adams[3] and B.J. Fogg for their amazing books on systems and goals respectively.

28 YOU CAN PUT EVERYTHING INTO A SEQUENCE

One of the most challenging aspects of being a human being is the non-stop flow of choices we must make each and every day. When I hear the alarm clock sounding in the morning I can choose to jump up or roll over and groan. When I haul myself out of the bed, I can choose to go to the shower straight away or I can amble downstairs and mooch around the kitchen. I can choose to swap my pajamas for clothes, or I can leave the pajamas on for the first hour of the day. And so on. There are so many choices. This choosing requires neural effort, like a cost to the brain.

It's the same set of choices when it comes to exercise. I can make it so that every day I have a set of choices to make, costing me precious neural energy and time, or I can do pretty much the same thing every day avoiding the need to choose and saving me time and effort. Most people have heard the story about Barack Obama wearing the same kind of clothes each day to avoid wasting time choosing at the wardrobe each morning. Steve Jobs did a similar thing for the same reason it seems. So, I have formed my mornings into something like a steady-state sequence that I tend to stick to most days.

I got the idea from the book Tiny Habits by B.J. Fogg. In the book (highly recommended) B.J. explains that by putting things into a system they become a lot more automatic and we are therefore more likely to stick with them like a habit we don't want to change. So, when I thought about my morning, I decided to create this sequence, or system as B.J. calls it, so that I would be more likely to stick with it, and boy did it work.

The night before I lay out my walking attire. Shirt, light fleece, rain jacket (if I expect rain), socks, shorts, jogging pants, shoes, watch, hat (or cap), sunglasses, and wireless earphones. When my alarm goes off, I get dressed in my exercise clothes right away. I don't face any resistance. There are no 'where are my damn shoes' moments to derail me. I get dressed and there's no going back now. I power on my earphones and pair them with my phone. I put them on my head, place my sunglasses on next, then my cap. Then downstairs where I do the same two things every day. I drink some water from the filter jug, grab my house keys from the kitchen and I quietly let myself out. Outside the front door I start my work out on my watch, fire up whatever podcast or audiobook I'm listening to, and I start my walk.

I stick to the same route every weekday, and the same weekend route when I'm out walking on Saturday and Sunday. I speak about why this is in another chapter, but you can surely see how not needing to choose a new route every day makes sense.

When I get back home after the walk I go to the kitchen and power off my headphones and remove my cap. I leave them aside while I drink more water. Then I grab my headphones and cap and bring them back upstairs, putting them where I expect to find them the next day. This is key, putting things in the same place every time makes it effortless to locate them.

The next part I added based on B.J. Fogg's book. He suggested that it's possible to work out every day if you bolt it on right before some other everyday activity, such as when you go to the shower. As I described in an earlier chapter, I figured because I just walked 5 km my muscles are nicely warmed up, so I added a step between getting home from the walk and stepping into the shower. With my exercise clothes still on I do a set of push-ups, a set of crunches and the same exercises with my 5kg dumbbell weights every time I walk. Because I do them as a matter of routine, because they are in the sequence, I almost always do them before I get to the shower.

I started out with just 5 push-ups because I was out of shape, but nowadays I usually do 15. I could do more, but I find that's enough to keep me feeling good. I'm not looking to set a personal best, as I've said before. Just enough exercise to make me feel good about it without causing me to hate my walk routine.

I then get on the floor and do my crunches, usually 15 but sometimes as many as 35.

That brings me to the weights. I bought these some time ago, a pair of 5 kg dumbbell weights. I don't even know what the exercises are called but I do three sets of 15 exercises. They give my arms a decent workout without the pain that I know will make me hate exercising so I'm happy with that. Some days I decide to add in one or two new things but these three, push-ups – crunches – weights, work just great for me. Then it's into the shower.

Believe it or not, I have created a routine for my shower too. Always doing things in the same sequence saves time and mental effort. Drying and applying moisturizer, combing hair, deodorant etc. is all done in sequence every day. Try it. You'll see that it just allows this to all flow so much easier with little or no choosing or deciding required.

Finally, when I am dressed, I head to the kitchen for eggs and coffee. Yes, that's done in a sequence too and it means it's one less thing to waste time thinking about.

There's no choosing or deliberating. I know what I am doing, and I just do it.

Putting things into a repeatable sequence is amazing, and if you have any concern that you might waver in your aim of becoming healthy and sticking with it, this is the way to go.

One final comment here from me about the exercises when I get home. These exercises work for me but if you have any history of injuries or pain it would make sense for you to do what's right for you, including discussing your plans with your doctor. Don't feel you need to do what I do. Identify what could work for you and keep adjusting until you're enjoying the routine and you are pain-free.

29 SWITCH TO ANOTHER REPEATABLE ROUTINE

If you create a single perfect routine, it makes things really easy to remember. The same order of getting dressed. The same order of exercises. The same order of drinking water before and after you exercise. The same route when you walk. But what happens if something upsets one small element of that order? What happens if that disruption lasts for more than a few days? What happens if someone you know asks if they can walk with you and wants to meet you somewhere near where they live to join up?

Don't get so attached to the idea of one perfect routine, because sooner or later you might need to make a tweak. Why not have at least one alternative routine that you can switch to without too much trouble and without causing everything to be messed up in your head.

Instead of leaving your home and turning right like always, why not allow for the possibility that one day you might need to turn left and complete the same route in the opposite direction. The idea here is not variety or novelty. That's not really adding anything. The idea is to allow you to still get your exercise without one thing blocking everything for a day or a few days. Sticking to a typical routine every day still makes huge sense but be flexible enough that you can change it up if you need to.

Maybe it's not the walk but it's a pre-exercise routine. For me, this is true when I think of what I plan to wear when I exercise outside. In summer I have a repeatable routine that eliminates any time wasted choosing what to wear. I know what my clothing options are, and I set what I want to wear out each night before I go walking. But when the cold weather comes, I switch to a new routine because I need to wear something warmer. My summer t-shirts go into storage and now I am preparing clothes that are appropriate for much colder weather. When spring comes and the weather gets milder these clothes will be put into storage and my t-shirts and shorts will become the routine again.

The same logic applies. Make it a routine so you know what to do and don't have time to change your mind or resist when exercise is the right thing to do and will be great for getting the day off to a good start. But don't just have one routine. Recognise when you need to switch to a new routine but make sure you have enough supplies of clothes or whatever will allow you to stick to the new routine for at least 3 days before laundry is an issue and you have nothing to wear.

30 EXERCISING WHEN LIFE MOVES YOU AWAY FROM HOME

Establishing your routine makes exercising every day much easier and a habit you are likely to maintain. So, what happens if you are required to be away from home for a few days? Long-distance travel that requires an overnight stay can really mess up your healthy exercise habit if you don't have a plan. So here's what I do when I have to travel or expect to be away from home for an extended period.

First, I pack a sports bag with all my exercise gear. My shoes, my clothes, my weights. Basically, everything that's portable and light and that will make me more likely to get some form of exercise while away. If I can't walk or jog but know that the place I'm going to has a swimming pool I'll pack my swimming shorts and a cap. If you don't have gear with you it's almost impossible for you to get any useful exercise while away.

If I'm planning to be away for a few days, then I expand the number of items I need so that I have what I need for each day I expect to be away. I don't expect to be doing any laundry while away, so I bring enough such that I have what I need every day.

If my trip involves a flight and I don't want to have to check a bag into the hold of the aircraft, I'll bring the bare minimum for exercise, but I'll still make a point of packing what I need.

My options when away are limited, but there are several options for a simple form of exercise. Since walking and some basic workout exercises are my normal routine, I instantly consider a walk of about 5km from wherever I am staying. I'll tend to check this out beforehand on google maps.

You can also use an app and plugin where you are and how far you want to walk, and it will help you devise a walk that meets your requirements. Once I am back from my walk, I will then be able to do some of my favourite exercises (push-ups, stretches etc.) in the hotel room before hitting the shower.

The second option is to use a hotel gym or local gym. I'm not a fan of gyms and am not a member of a gym anywhere. If this works well for you and the gym has some equipment that you like and are happy to use, then this should be a viable option. Again, stretching and exercising on your own in your room afterwards is possible.

The third option, especially if you're in a place that's super cold or potentially dangerous outside, is to exercise in your room. You might not be able to walk for 5km, but you can certainly do some exercise, and that's my golden rule right there. If you can't do everything then just do something. Any amount of any exercise is better than no exercise at all.

If you like to swim and there is a pool in your hotel or nearby that's a decent option if you can swim. It might make exercising in the room afterwards impractical though, especially if you take a shower right after your swim.

No matter where you are there is something you can do when it comes to exercise. Remember though that when away for work it's common to eat larger meal portions, to snack more regularly on junk, and to drink more coffee and sugary drinks and less water. All of this will undermine the benefits of some basic exercise.

Try to consciously only eat as much as you need. Manage your snacking and have your own snacks with you if that helps to avoid chocolate and sugary treats. Set a limit on how much coffee you want in the day and try not to drink any caffeinated coffee after dinner time. And plenty of water. Lots of water.

31 ANY AMOUNT OF ANY EXERCISE - EVERY DAY

For me, the worst thing I could do would be to create a routine that feels like hardship. I don't want to wake up each day and hear my mind think "I suppose I'd better do this now or I'll feel guilty later".

I want to feel good about going for a walk, listening to a book or podcast, getting some clean air into my lungs and gently working the muscles in my body. I know that anything I do that creates a negative association won't make me more likely to exercise. It will become a turn off that could cause me to stop exercising altogether.

So, I don't get too hung up on routine, at least not to the extent that I worry if I break the sequence of daily walks. I understand that some days I just can't get out for a walk. My work schedule on a certain day might have me starting work very early, so early that it's not feasible to fit in some exercise before I get down to work. Other days might go on so long that it's almost 9 pm when I'm finishing up my last video call or online meeting.

On days like these, I satisfy myself that I did all I could do, and it might not be much. But it does need to be something by way of exercise, even if it's just 5 minutes of effort. So, I might do a set of exercises just before getting into bed. Not enough that I'm sweating in bed but enough that I have worked some muscles. Maybe some push-ups, followed by some crunches followed by some work with the dumbbell weights I keep in the bedroom. If I can't do that, maybe I'll take the dog for a short walk, or I'll do some tidying and moving stuff about to put things in order.

The key point here is that there is more than one way to exercise. The key is to get some exercise, any exercise. It's not so crucial that it's different to what I did yesterday or that it's not helping me keep my apple watch happy. That's not important at all. Do what you can, every day.

You'll have better days and maybe even better weeks, but some days you can't do what you hoped. In these moments, do something else instead of your usual routine, but don't do nothing. Don't fall into a habit of making exercise a thing you do only when everything else falls perfectly into place. That will make exercise an occasional thing you do which is not going to help you at all.

Keep moving, keep active, keep looking for ways in which you can incorporate a little bit of exercise when the ideal is not available. Take the stairs instead of the elevator. Walk a little bit faster than you normally would. Park a little further away to ensure you get a walk. Instead of sitting in your car at the school flicking through social media why not get a short walk in before the school finishes for the day.

Get creative and find a way to build in a little exercise every single day when you can. Some days it just won't happen but the days you don't get any exercise should be the exception. Look closer at the time you have. You'll find a way to include a little exercise every single day if you look closely enough.

32 SLEEP LIKE IT'S URGENT

The body and brain benefit from exercise. That much should be clear by now. Equally, eating well and hydrating sufficiently throughout the day are vital too. But what about sleep? Sleep is one of those areas that modern living seems to have corrupted and reframed as a variable-necessity. We broadly accept the need for sleep but seem to disagree about how much each of us needs in order to function properly.

The term "function properly" is problematic too. Different people will make the argument that by sleeping for as few as 2 or 3 hours a night they can function normally and do all the things they want and need to do in a day. They believe they can "function properly" on a tiny amount of sleep. Could this possibly be true? Are there millions or billions of us sleeping too long each night when a mere 2 or 3 hours is sufficient? Let me answer that right here. It's not true. Psychologist Dabiel Levitin's work shows clearly that we can't function properly on a mere 2 or 3 hours of sleep and expect to get through a day without there being problems with energy, concentration, decision making and a whole list of other daily necessities[4]. The body and brain can survive with a small amount of sleep but we're not at our best. Worse, over time this low sleep level will affect our health in a variety of ways and may even affect your eventual lifespan.

We need sleep and we need a good amount of sleep, because sleep is vital to bodily health and regeneration. The brain needs sleep at night so it can get to work doing what brains do when we sleep, namely categorizing and sorting what we experienced during the day and purging waste material back into the bloodstream via the blood-brain barrier.

When we don't sleep enough the brain can't file away learning and experiences properly, so memories might not work so well when we need to retrieve them. When we don't sleep enough the brain can't flush out the depleted blood supply and waste matter and replace it with fresh oxygenated blood needed to keep the brain working in peak condition.

The need for sleep feels intuitively right but seems to have become culturally wrong. Sleeping less and working more is often held up as a sign of commitment, drive, strength, or power. Those who sleep only a few hours a night claim to suffer no ill-effects, but this simply isn't true. We all need sleep to rest, recover and regenerate.

Yet we find consistently that we go to bed too late and get up in the morning to the sound of an alarm clock that pains us. "It can't be that time already!" is a familiar thought to millions of us, and it signals the onset of another day to be endured while pumped up on caffeine and sugar to hopefully propel us to the end of the working day.

While we can't change much about the time we need to wake up, we can prolong sleep by going to bed a little earlier. This option is available to almost all of us, yet we rarely take up this option. We try to cram ever more activity into our evenings, watching TV or Netflix or YouTube right to the moment where our eyes can stay open no more. We fall asleep only to wake up not feeling refreshed at all.

Sleep is vital and without the right amount there's little to be gained from exercising regularly and eating well. The body's needs will be out of balance, not to mention a generally fuzzy brain state. Instead of using our intelligence to make the case for going to bed early, we have wasted so many nights making the case for more TV or more internet surfing instead.

So, the challenge is this. Can you work out how much sleep you need so that you feel fully rested? Can you try for a week to work out what time you should switch off the light and close your eyes so that you feel great when you wake up the following morning? Take a notebook for the next 7 nights and try going to bed even 15 minutes earlier each night than the night before. Note in the book how you feel in the morning and see if you can come to a conclusion about how much sleep you need, and what time you should go to bed.

The other part to this is all about bedtime habits. If you keep your phone beside the bed is there a way you could leave it in another room for the first night and use an old-fashioned clock-radio or alarm clock to wake you up? Same deal for tablets and laptops and your smart watch. Another room each night to see if it plays a role in messing with your sleep. If you have a TV in the room it would be a good idea to leave the remote next to your phone in another room. You won't be tempted to use it and you'll know where to find it in the morning.

Sleep is seriously important, and we have been telling ourselves lies about how much we need and how strong we are without enough of it. Find a way to protect your sleep routine, like it's the most urgent thing you need to do at night.

Make a good night's sleep more urgent than your need to check the news headlines or catch up on some YouTube channel you follow. Your body and brain will thank you for it, and all that exercise and healthy eating will not be in vain.

33 MOTIVATIONAL COLLAPSE

We all have those periods where the motivation to do anything is completely gone. Some bad news, a nightmare day at work, a breach of trust, or any other number of possible causes and we just can't be bothered to carry on. It happens to everyone at some point. Don't beat yourself up.

Take the time you need and don't bully yourself into doing exercise or walking when your heart is not in it. Recognize that there could be some kind of internal war going on inside you. One inner voice is whispering guilty things into your ear. "I knew you'd quit. You always quit". The other voice is whispering competing messages into your other ear "you need to take a step back. This is a bad time." These voices are the kind of thing that creates a tense standoff in your own head.

Forget about choosing a voice. Do what you need to do to get through whatever is making you feel demotivated.

Be where you need to be. Just know that there's always room for a tiny step back to normal.

Even at your lowest ebb, the tiniest gesture sends a signal to your brain that you're coming back. Seriously. The tiniest gesture. Try this for example. If you can't bring yourself to walk 5 km today, or any day soon, make time for a standing-up push-up against the wall next time you go to the bathroom. One standing push-up. That's it. Or if you're tempted to eat the whole back of Doritos or pour out a huge bowl of sugary breakfast cereal – don't. Cut back a little. You'd be amazed what a little act like this signals to your brain. It's the inflection point. The point at the bottom of the curve where the curve down starts to turn back up.

Take it slow. There's no need to rush. If something is on your mind, then that's fine. But watch out for the moment when you can send a tiny signal to your brain that you're coming back. Take that step, send that tiny signal. And watch as you slowly start to rebuild your motivation again.

No matter how far down you have fallen, you really can start to climb back up with the tiniest starting step. Follow that first small amount of activity with another small amount on day 2, and you're already building some momentum.

34 MISSING A DAY

From time to time, unanticipated things happen, and you'll be forced to miss a day. Remember that exercise is your friend. Not your boss or schoolteacher wondering where you were yesterday. It's your body, and your exercise routine, so do what you need to do, and go where you are needed. Then when you're ready, go back to your exercise routine.

There's no point in beating yourself up when you miss a day. Even if you just don't feel like you have the energy, this is likely a sign from your body and brain that today would be a good day for some rest and recovery. The signals you get are important to heed so don't let guilt or shame force you to keep going when missing a day makes more sense.

This is one of the reasons why I prefer to exercise on my own rather than with a walking buddy or partner. I need to have the flexibility and don't want to be answerable to anyone else when things get in the way that I can't ignore.

Recently one of the children was referred by the family doctor for a COVID-19 test. He had a cough and a headache and a sore throat. The doctor said he should get tested so my wife took him to the test center. Protocol dictates that everyone else in the house should isolate until the test results come back, typically 24-48 hours later. I had no choice. I couldn't go out and walk, even though I was confident he didn't have COVID-19. 30 hours later the results came back, and he was clear. He did not have COVID-19.

The next morning, I was out for my morning walk. No big deal. No drama. Stuff happens. Take a day or two to do what you need to do. Then start again when you're ready.

35 WHEN ILLNESS STRIKES

We all get sick. It happens. We can't plan it nor can we rush ourselves back to health any faster than the body and modern medicine allows. So, when you get sick, watch out for the silly phase where your mind tells you that exercising when sick might actually help.

It's tempting to play the role of the amateur physician and decide that migraine or an earache isn't enough to throw you out of your routine. Are you sure about that? What if you're wrong and you end up making a not so bad situation into a worse situation. Exercising with a migraine is a good example. You'll probably regret doing that for some time.

If you are ill, your body will find a clever way to let you know. Usually, you'll feel like hell and want to crash on the sofa or in bed until you feel human again. This is a clever mechanism that our evolutionary biology has devised to stop us from doing harm when we're ill.

Take a few days, or whatever you need. If you can still walk up and down the stairs at home, that's still exercise. If you're moving muscles by reaching up or down to find your medicine or hot water blanket that's exercise. Every little helps when you're ill.

And if you're too ill to do even that, then give yourself a break and allow yourself the time to heal. Recovery is one of the most important aspects of living a healthy life. Rushing back to work or sport or whatever before you are ready is a bad idea and disrespects the work that your body and brain are doing to make you well again.

When you are ill, take a break from the normal routine. Get some advice, follow that advice, and rest according to what the body needs in order to recover fully. Don't be tempted to think you know better and shave off 20% to 50% of the recovery time. That's one surefire way to guarantee that you'll still have the remnants of an illness long after you should.

Be kind to yourself means giving yourself the right time, the right care, and the right rest when you're ill. When you're over your illness your walking shoes and exercise clothes will be ready to go. Everything will wait for you until you're healthy again.

36 STORMY WEATHER

You can control a great many things in your life but not everything. It can feel very important to stick to your exercise routine. Waking at the same time and putting on your exercise clothes in the same sequence sends a signal of commitment and forged habit to your brain. It can be strange when a thought flashes across your mind that maybe you won't go for a walk today. If the reason you have a thought that tempts you to miss your daily walk is just laziness or low drive, then you should push past that and stick with your walking commitment.

If, however, the reason you think you won't go for your walk today is because some really bad weather is forecast then that's different. Seriously different. Your body and brain will always benefit from exercise and will thank you for a walk in fresh clean air. But your body and brain won't thank you if you expose them to real harm or the risk of injury because you simply don't want to break a commitment. As a rule, I never go out to exercise if there is a chance of bad weather. I don't mean light rain. That's fine. But heavy rain will be enough for me to change up my exercise approach. Instead of an early morning walk, I'll either walk on the treadmill for the same distance at another time in the day or will find some other way to get some amount of exercise, even if it's less than I'd get by walking.

If there is very cold weather forecast that's much more serious. You could slip and really injure yourself. Sure, you're the kind of person that is careful. That would never happen to you. Is it really worth the risk for the sake of exercise when you could exercise in some way at home until the weather improves? That's my approach and so far, so good on the no serious injury score. You could also meet the dangerous coming together of you hot and sweaty in your clothes meeting very cold air temperature. This is when frostbite or hypothermia could strike you.

I don't exercise outdoors when the weather threatens me and could cause me harm. The idea, once again, is to make exercise a thing that makes you feel great and is something to look forward to every day. If the result of your exercise in extreme weather is a sprained ankle, pneumonia, frostbite, or hypothermia then you really won't feel great and you'll have done the one thing I strive to avoid at all costs. Making any kind of negative association with exercise will make you less likely to want it in your daily life. Keep exercise fun, enjoyable and flexible. Make it work with you and for you.

37 RISKING IT ALL FOR A WALK

I turned 50 in the year 2020. A memorable year for various reasons, not least the arrival into the world of the COVID-19 pandemic. Initially where I live there were some restrictions on the grounds of protecting public health. Schools and businesses were closed to try and curtail the spread of the virus.

This helped me initially to carve out time for a walk each morning before starting my online work. This coincided with good weather and generally quiet roads each morning. It was the ideal conditions for walking.

As the year progressed the virus seemed to ebb and flow around the world, one moment looking like things were getting back under control before wildly getting out of control again. Recently the virus is on the rise again and case numbers are escalating rapidly. Public health measures have been reimposed to limit people from moving about more than is absolutely necessary.

I am conflicted about my walking routine as I write. I want to walk, and the conditions are good, but there is a general call for people to stay home and avoid contact with one another for the next little while.

I started walking because I knew it would be good for my health. My improved health would be good for my family and our future together. I walk because it's simple and safe and poses no real threat to my body as long as I don't overdo it with the distance or pace I set. If I decide to continue walking while this virus is actively spreading, I am putting my health at risk. It might be low risk but it's a risk I don't need to take right now. If I put myself at risk, I also put my family at risk. The entire rationale for my walks centers around improving my health in a low to no risk way. That's not what walking right now represents.

So, here's what I'm going to do. I'm pausing my walks for the time being. I will do other activities instead. I'll use the treadmill even though it's not the same. I will do some exercises. I will make sure to find reasons to use the stairs as often as I can. Maybe I'll even get on the exercise bike again for a while.

If I can give myself a little exercise and activity for the next little while, and at the same time limit my exposure to the risk of contracting COVID-19 that makes the most sense to me.

I know there will be others who want to press ahead and keep exercising near others. You do whatever you think is best. I'm going to stay true to why I started walking in the first instance.

It's not a race. I don't need to risk everything to honor my routine. I will adapt for the time being, just like I would if the weather was very bad, and when it's time to re-engage in my 5 km walk on my usual route, that's where I'll be as soon as it's safe to do so.

One final point about walking and exercise in a time of pandemic. While you need to protect yourself and your health, and by extension protect the health and safety of your loved ones, you do need to consider the possibility that your exercise might cause danger or distress to others.

If you must exercise, do so within the guidance set out by your local health authority. Don't be tempted to brush this off as over the top worrying by people who don't understand. Don't be tempted to sell yourself the idea that exercise is necessary at all costs. Be responsible to yourself and to your fellow citizens.

38 UNDOING ALL YOUR GOOD WORK

You already know that even the simple act of a regular walk will make you feel healthier. Throw in some light exercises and more attention to things you eat and drink and your body will already start showing signs of better health.

You also know that better health comes from replacing bad habits with good habits. Making sure you get at least 7 hours of sleep a night, as often as you can, will help. Eating less junk food and eating appropriate portions will help. Walking for between 30 and 60 minutes a day will help. Taking the stairs instead of the elevator or escalator will help. Drinking plenty of water and avoiding things that will cause you stress – they'll help too.

It doesn't take much to undo all your good work. A drop in motivation, a period of time away from home especially if you are alone, or any number of other setbacks or upsets could really throw you off balance. This can bring out the rebellious child in all of us and we may turn to the very things we know are bad for us. Staying up all night and not getting sufficient sleep. Overeating on junk and other unhealthy food. Too much alcohol or sugary drinks. No exercise whatsoever and not enough water consumed each day. Before you know if you will be in a bad state. It can easily happen.

Any one of these can be problematic, but more than one at once and you can slip into bad health really fast. Sometimes just being around other people can unsettle us without us really noticing. The conversation has become filled with anger and injustice. The system is rigged. It's not fair. Someone has screwed you out of something that's rightfully yours. Often being with other people can anchor us in a place where we feel no option than to join in with the bitching and complaining. Joining in with the binge eating and drinking, staying up late and not sleeping enough, and so on.

Your good work is for you. It should make you feel healthy and in control of your own day and how you feel throughout that day. Sometimes when you feel things starting to slip out of control it might be worth trying to clear some space for yourself to weigh up what's happening and why.

We all have down periods where things aren't fun and where the temptation to give in is loud and near. But you already know what to do. You already have the formula to get out of that dip and to start feeling healthy and in control again. Go back to the beginning and remind yourself how you began. Maybe it was that single push up, or that first 5-minute outdoor walk. This is where the answer lies.

No amount of escaping through drinking or eating or whatever it is that you hope will numb you to life can hide what's going on forever. If there's something eating at you and you need to talk to someone about that then you should do that soon. Unattended issues rarely resolve themselves by ignoring them. Tackle what's undermining you and stay grounded in the real world. Notice which people are good for you right now and will help you to feel good and healthy again. Notice which people are not good for you and want to drag you down to escape reality and numb yourself from your problem.

Do what's right for you and steer back towards what feels positive, healthy, and gives you the energy that you need so that you wake up each morning ready to make the best of each day.

39 CONCLUSION: BE KIND TO YOURSELF

Why bother with being healthy? Who cares, right? Well, if you care about yourself, or live with other family members who care about you, you should care about your health.

Having witnessed at first hand a family member suffer with extreme health problems after a life of not caring about his health, it's a terrible thing to witness. To see someone that was healthy, vibrant, and enjoying life start to slip into poor health, eventually not able to do even the most basic things, it's awful. Nobody should want that for themselves or for those who care about them.

Take responsibility for how you feel every day. Your health is yours to mind and care for and you should treat your health as a precious gift. And if the aim is to be healthy and to stay healthy, then what your body demands of you is quite simple and quite basic.

Don't put too much bad stuff inside. Go easy on foods and liquids that are not good for you in big quantities. Every extra unit consumed is a battle the body must wage. Think about how much of the "I know it's bad for me but I like it" stuff you consume and aim to cut back, even a little at a time. It will really help your health in the long run.

Put plenty of the good stuff inside. Foods that are natural, close to their original state as they were picked, dug up, fished out of the sea, or whatever way they ended up in your shopping cart – these will be one of the gifts you give to your body and brain. Vegetables, fruit, nuts, seeds, fish, and meat (in appropriate forms) are things that the body can work with. They take longer to digest, unlike processed foods, but they don't end up causing an internal war with your body and brain.

Sleep is also a gift. Telling yourself you don't need it is a lie. A deception that so many of us try to perpetrate upon ourselves is that we are capable of coping with 4 or 5 hours of sleep. That's survival talk. Thriving, doing well, feeling at optimal health – that needs more sleep. 7 to 8 hours is recommended for good reason, not least because the body and brain need that long to reset during the night and wash out the waste in the bloodstream from the day before.

The final gift is exercise. Exercise keeps things flexible, functional, and ready for work. When we tell ourselves that the best way to spend every evening is on the couch with a beer, that every sunny evening is an evening to fire up the grill for a meat feast, that every spare few hours is the time to sit on the sideline at a sports event eating and drinking. These are all choices we can make, and the key is the word "every".

Life needs balance. Health needs balance. You need balance. Find time to exercise and your body and brain will benefit greatly. Invest your thinking power in excuse-making for why you don't need exercise and your body and brain will wither. Maybe not noticeably at first but give it time and before long getting off the sofa will take grunting and groaning. You'll notice you're not so sharp anymore at remembering the name of that guy in that film.

Exercise keeps things working well. Not for Olympic-level exertion but for life. Exercise sounds optional but it really shouldn't be. It's your choice and you can choose how often to get out and do something good for your body and your brain.

Doing nothing every day is a golden ticket to the kind of health collapse that I personally witnessed, that I would not wish on anyone ever. Do it now while you can. Make tonight the night you walk for 10 minutes. Or tomorrow the first 20-minute walk you have taken while everyone else is still sleeping.

Whatever you do, don't do nothing. Be kind to yourself. Keep active and keep exercising while you can. You'll be forever grateful that you did.

EXTRA RESOURCES FOR YOU

If you would like to see the details of my warm weather or cold weather daily routines, you can find them on the Facebook page for this book. Search for Healthy at Fifty or click the following link to go to the Facebook page:

https://www.facebook.com/Healthy-at-Fifty-101192468632842/

You can download details of my routines. You can also edit them to create your own daily routine until it becomes a habit that you have learned off by heart.

You can also find information about recommended clothes, shoes, and any other items that I mentioned in the book. These are items I would happily recommend to you based on my own experience of ownership and use.

I also will post regular updates and short posts with links to useful articles. If you would like to be notified when these new items are published, you can subscribe to my page so you don't miss anything in the months ahead.

Thanks for reading all the way to the end. I hope you found this book useful and interesting and I wish you the very best health every day from here.

Sincere thanks my friend,

Justin.

ABOUT THE AUTHOR

JUSTIN KINNEAR is the author of *The Small Business Advantage: From Surviving to Thriving Through Outstanding Customer Service* and *The Nine Signs of Saying Goodbye*.

He lives in Ireland with his wife and two sons.

Justin writes to share his favourite learning and experiences, and to inspire others to explore possibilities that they have never noticed before.

OTHER BOOKS BY JUSTIN G. KINNEAR

The Nine Signs Of Saying Goodbye (Kindle edition)

The Small Business Advantage: From Surviving to Thriving Through Outstanding Customer Service

BOOKS MENTIONED IN THE TEXT

Throughout this book I have made reference to some other excellent books that I enjoyed and that helped me to create a new and sustainable walking routine. Here are the details of those books in case you would like to check them out.

---

[1] The Source: The Secrets of the Universe, The Science of the Brain, by Dr. Tara Swart,

[2] Tiny Habits: The Small Changes That Change Everything, by Dr. B.J. Fogg PhD

[3] How to Fail at Almost Everything and Still Win Big: Kind of the Story of My Life, by Scott Adams

[4] The Organized Mind: Thinking Straight in the Age of Information Overload, by Daniel Levitin